Hyperthyroidism Cure

*The Most Effective, Permanent
Solution To Finally Overcome
Hyperthyroidism For Life*

Elizabeth Grace

Table of Content

Conclusion

Introduction

The human body is like a giant company whose success and productivity depend on the cooperation of hundreds of departments. Overseeing much of this cooperation is the endocrine system; a group of organs whose job is to make hormones--chemical messengers that travel throughout the body in the bloodstream.

Let's talk about one in particular: the Thyroid. The thyroid is a butterfly-shaped organ located in the lower neck. Control of the thyroid starts in the brain at an area called the Hypothalamus. Using hormones of its own, the Hypothalamus sends a signal to a gland called the Pituitary, causing it to release Thyroid Stimulating Hormone or TSH.

TSH travels through the bloodstream until it gets to the thyroid. Stimulated by TSH, the thyroid releases two hormones: T3 and T4 (Thyroxine). Together, these are known simply as thyroid hormones. Thyroid hormones have many important functions in the body. They control how fast your body uses the energy in the food you eat.

Aside from that, they control body temperature, the way muscles contract, and increase your heart rate to name a few. Now, the amount of hormone released by the thyroid is crucial. It is similarly important to how much water you give a plant. Water it too little and it will shrivel up. Water it too much and it will drown. However, with just the right amount, you get a happy and healthy plant.

Your body is the same way. Without enough thyroid hormone, things start to go wrong. We call this, Hypothyroidism. It is characterized by symptoms like fatigue, weight gain, thinning hair, and depression.

Too much thyroid hormone can also cause problems. This is known as Hyperthyroidism. So what causes Hyperthyroidism? Well, according to the AAFP (American Academy of Family Physicians), the most common cause of Hyperthyroidism is a disease called Grave's disease. In fact, it is responsible for about 50-80% of all cases usually seen in women between the ages of 30 to 50. This disease is seen 4-10 times more in women than in men.

This book will talk about Hyperthyroidism and Grave's disease in-depth. We will talk about their underlying causes and other possible risk factors. Not only that, this book will also talk about natural therapies and supplements that you can take to get rid of Hyperthyroidism for life.

So, sit back and relax and let your journey of healing from Hyperthyroidism begin.

Chapter 1: What is Hyperthyroidism?

So what is Hyperthyroidism? Hyperthyroidism is basically the elevation of the thyroid hormone. Thyroid hormones basically come in two forms: The T3 and T4 thyroid hormones. Most T3 and T4 are bound to thyroid binding globulin or TBG, which renders them inactive. There are, however, T3 and T4 thyroid hormone that are not bound to TBG. These are called "free" T3 or T4. Between the two thyroid hormones, T3 is the one that is more active.

Hyperthyroidism has two types, the Primary hyperthyroidism, and Secondary hyperthyroidism.

- Primary hyperthyroidism - This is generally where most kinds of hyperthyroidism fall under. Primary hyperthyroidism is characterized by an elevated thyroid hormone that's due to increased production by the thyroid for one reason or another. In this case, the thyroid is creating too much thyroid hormone and is the reason why a person has hyperthyroidism. Remember, hyperthyroidism is basically about an overproduction of thyroid hormone. It has nothing to do with any other factors whatsoever.

Because you're going to have a high T3 and a high T4, you're therefore going to have a low thyroid-stimulating hormone or TSH. Having low TSH will also, in turn, give you a negative feedback.

- Secondary hyperthyroidism - The hyperthyroidism is considered secondary because of the elevated TSH. In this case, you have stimulation of the thyroid by TSH and that's why it is called secondary hyperthyroidism. While you still have high T3 and high T4, you have elevated TSH because the cause is actually the elevated TSH. Here, you will have negative feedback and that you have elevated TSH as the cause.

An example of secondary hyperthyroidism would be Pituitary Adenoma. The symptoms of hyperthyroidism are going to be the same regardless of whether it is primary or secondary hyperthyroidism. Examples of these symptoms would be nervousness, emotional liability, tremor, insomnia, sweating, heat intolerance, weight loss, increased appetite, palpitations--which can be a sign of atrial fibrillation--warm and moist skin, menstrual changes, and hypercalcemia. Hypercalcemia is actually due to the fact that thyroid hormones activate osteoclast activity.

When you suspect hyperthyroidism, or hypothyroidism for that matter, the best initial test is going to be TSH. That will rule it in or rule it out right away. If by any chance you're a doctor and you have a patient with hyperthyroidism indeed, then you should have a high T3 and T4 and either low or high TSH. Provided that the patient is stable, the best initial test is to get a TSH.

Hyperthyroidism: Differential Diagnosis

Primary hyperthyroidism (high T3 and T4, low TSH) - Just like what we have discussed earlier, the only characteristic that primary hyperthyroidism share with secondary hyperthyroidism is the high T3 and T4. Its difference from secondary hyperthyroidism is that fact that it has low TSH.

Secondary hyperthyroidism (high T3 and T4, high TSH) – The only difference of Secondary hyperthyroidisms from its primary counterpart is that it has a high TSH.

- Pheochromocytoma - Pheochromocytoma is basically a tumor of the adrenal gland that secretes epinephrine. In this case, you're going to have an extremely elevated blood pressure. This doesn't happen much in hyperthyroidism. You may make it to tachycardia with hyperthyroidism, however, you're not going to have a severely elevated blood pressure.

- Acute manic episode - Acute manic episode can present similar symptoms to hyperthyroidism. However, in acute manic episodes, you're going to be limited to the psychiatric symptoms of hyperthyroidism. For instance, nervousness, tremor, insomnia, etc. but you're not going to have changes in appetite; you're not going to have weight loss, you're not going to have palpitations, and so forth.

- Cocaine intoxication - Cocaine intoxication can present similar symptoms to hyperthyroidism such as nervousness, fatigue, insomnia. However, you're not going to have weight loss or menstrual changes.

- Amphetamine intoxication - Amphetamine is fairly similar to cocaine intoxication when it comes to differential diagnosis with hyperthyroidism.

What Is an Autoimmune Disease?

There are many complicated and confusing explanations for this. However, the most simple and accurate explanation is that it's an immune system confusion problem. In certain ways, your immune system is overreacting and making antibodies that attack your own body.

The immune system has lost the capability to tell friendly from non-friendly cells. Also, the immune system is under-functioning and it won't be taking care of invaders and other things that it is supposed to take care of.

Autoimmune Disease Triggers

One trigger of this immune system confusion is a mechanism called "*Molecular Mimicry*," which is closely tied to gastrointestinal health. The surface area of our digestive system--specifically the small intestines--is about the size of a tennis court. And across this entire surface area, the digestive system and immune system is working to make sure that we don't have too many things come into the body that really shouldn't.

One of the things that we do not want to enter our body is an Antigen. Antigens could be food that we're allergic to, microbes, bacteria, fungus, basically anything the immune system needs to target and eliminate. Before these antigens are able to completely enter our body, they first have to go through what's called a mucus layer. This mucus layer is where antigens pass through--a border of sorts-- before the immune system can target them.

Usually, the mucosal layer is really tight and prevents most antigens from entering the body. In *Molecular Mimicry*, however, the mucosal layer is loose. With a loose mucosal layer, antigens are able to enter the body easily.

This loosening of the gastrointestinal mucosal layer is what's called a "Leaky gut." The immune system, overwhelmed with all these antigens, in turn, starts making a lot of antibodies. These antibodies will attack and eliminate these antigens that are able to enter the body.

The problem with this is that some antigens may in some way look like your own cells. And due to your immune system's haste to eliminate the increased influx of antigens in your body, it will now have a hard time differentiating antigens from friendly cells. Coupled with the increased production of antibodies, there is now a high possibility that you have an autoimmune disease.

Molecular Mimicry is actually a trigger for many autoimmune diseases. Keep in mind that we just went through the signs in a simplified way. The key concept is that we have a compromised mucosal layer and immune system that is being overly triggered by certain microbes or antigens in the digestive tract.

3 Factors for Molecular Mimicry

The three factors that we need for Molecular Mimicry to occur are:

1. Genetic susceptibility - This is not a genetic disease. If you don't have the other factors, you're not going to get it. Genetic susceptibility does not mean genetic inevitability. Too many times things are blamed on genetics that just simply should not be.

2. Immune system trigger - This can be gluten, which we're going to get into in the succeeding chapters, or it can be some dysbiotic organisms.

3. Compromised border - This is another factor that must be present. Why? Because if you can't get something into the body for the immune system to react to, then you're not going to get the autoimmune response.

Grave's Disease

People and medical experts alike believe that Grave's disease is the primary cause of hyperthyroidism. It is a thyroid disease that is autoimmune in origin. And just like other autoimmune diseases, Grave's disease is also prevalent in women. The ratio at which Grave's disease infects women is 7-8:1.

In the case of Grave's disease, what you have is a circulating immunoglobulin--an antibody that's actually stimulating the TSH receptors. Because of that, you have a thyroid that's just basically active all the time regardless of whether or not you're secreting higher or lower levels of TSH.

You have an immunoglobulin that's constantly stimulating the thyroid. And so, you're going to have a low TSH level because you will have negative feedback. The immunoglobulins are not TSH. They are actually antibodies that are glycoprotein in nature that is produced by the body's plasma cell, or what we call our white blood cells.

Immunoglobulins are an essential part of your body's immune system. They have the ability to recognize and bind to particular antigens in our body, such as viruses or bacteria and assist in their elimination.

As mentioned, Grave's disease is more prevalent in women and the age of onset tends to fall between 20 to 40 years of age. Grave's disease, like other autoimmune diseases, is associated with other autoimmune disorders. If you're a doctor, you may have a patient with brain disease that also happens to have rheumatoid arthritis, or lupus.

Along with the hyperthyroid symptoms that we already mentioned, Grave's disease is notoriously associated with ocular symptoms such as Ophthalmoplegia and Exophthalmos. Ophthalmoplegia is characterized by paralysis or sense of pain when moving the eye muscles. Exophthalmos, on the other hand, is what most doctors call a bulging eye. Grave's disease is also associated with a dermatologic symptom known as pre-tibial myxedema, which is an induration and erythema of the skin over the shin.

Grave's Disease Triggers

One potential trigger of Grave's disease seems to be a bacterium called Yersinia enterocolitica, which can live in the gastrointestinal system. Countless medical studies have shown that people with Grave's disease have antibodies against Yersinia. On the other hand, people without Grave's disease, have none.

Another microbe which seems connected to Grave's disease is H. Pylori, which is more commonly known for its association with some gastric ulcers. There's a study way back in 1998 showing H. Pylori connected to autoimmune thyroid diseases including Hashimoto's disease and Grave's disease.

While we have medical studies showing the relationship of the aforementioned triggers of Grave's disease, the knowledge gathered from these studies do not make their way into standard medical practice; the knowledge is not used to directly treat the triggers and prevent the actual disease. Instead, most physicians will just recommend the destruction of the thyroid. There are, however, natural therapies that are designed to deal with H. Pylori, Yersinia, and other dysbiotic organisms.

Symptoms of Grave's Disease

The symptoms of Grave's disease are going to include your typical symptoms of hyperthyroidism: pre-tibial myxedema, menstrual changes, palpitations, increased appetite, insomnia, visual changes, sensitivity to heat, goiter, weight loss, and nervousness. Also, keep in mind that any disease that cause hyperthyroidism will also cause goiter. Why? Because it is causing an increased production of thyroid hormone.

When giving a patient afflicted with Grave's disease a physical examination, do not forget to take note of the increased heart rate, goiter, warm and moist skin, and fine tremors. If you're only suspecting Grave's disease, the most accurate test is going to be a serology for thyroid-stimulating immunoglobulin. If that comes back positive, it's diagnostic of Grave's disease.

Treatment of Grave's Disease

The treatment for Grave's disease is really two-fold: Treating the symptoms and treating the disease. To treat the symptoms, we use the selective beta-blocker propranolol, which is considered to be the best beta-blocker. As far as treating Grave's disease itself, we can go one of two routes. We can either use medical therapy, or we can do definitive therapy.

Using medical therapy to treat Grave's disease would involve the use of two anti-thyroid drugs: Propylthriouracil and Methimazole. Definitive therapy, on the other hand, is going to be injecting the patient with radioiodine. Radioiodine is actually going to destroy the thyroid altogether.

The only time we don't want to use radioiodine is in pregnant women or children. In most cases, however, we're going to just administer PTU and then do the radioiodine ablation to patients when it's appropriate.

If we want to treat Grave's disease medically in patients who are pregnant or who are children, we're going to use Propylthriouracil (PTU). Keep in mind that we're going to use PTU in pregnant women, not Methimazole. Why? Because Methimazole may cross the placenta and cause congenital defects in the fetus. We can also do surgery on pregnant women or children. If we do surgery, we would do a subtotal thyroidectomy.

The only time you can do a radioiodine ablation is after the woman delivers her baby. If you really have to do a definitive therapy to a pregnant woman or a child, then the definitive therapy would be subtotal thyroidectomy.

Chapter 2: Leaky gut and Dysbiosis

Aside from using natural therapies to kill dysbiotic organisms that can cause autoimmune diseases, we can also use natural therapies for the *Leaky gut*. *Leaky gut*, also called gut hyperpermeability, is a weakness in the digestive system's mucosal membranes which allows things to get through that shouldn't. This exposes the immune system to too many antigens.

Too many antigens coming from the digestive tract often leads to immune system confusion. This is common in many autoimmune diseases, whether it's Grave's disease, Hashimoto's disease, psoriasis, rheumatoid arthritis, etc.

Herbs and Supplements for Leaky Gut

There are so many supplements that can address a Leaky gut in the event that it becomes an issue. Here are some examples:

1. L-glutamine

2. N-acetyl-glucosamine

3. MSN

4. Herbs

5. Quercitin

6. Okra

7. Marshmallow

8. DGL licorice

9. Cat's claw

10. Chamomile

11. Slippery elm

There are many supplements that can treat a Leaky gut. The ones mentioned above are considered by many physicians as effective natural treatments for not only a Leaky gut, but also other autoimmune diseases.

Toxicity and Auto-immune Disease

Aside from looking at the gastrointestinal and microbial factors related to autoimmune diseases, you also need to consider someone's entire medical history in relation to toxicity. Is there a history of possible heavy metal exposure? What is going on in their work or home environment? What about dental work? Is there any possibility that a sub-acute infection occurred?

We want to look for things that can disrupt immune system function. In addition, we need to look at the patient's antibiotic history as that can also disrupt overall immune system function. If the case leads to more of an issue of toxicity and the need to detoxify, then that's where the case goes. With Grave's disease-- or any autoimmune disease for that matter--there is no "one-size-fits-all" etiology.

You must look at each autoimmune disease case differently. You must observe what the person's body is trying to do, what his or her health challenges are, etc. in order to normalize immune system function.

Immune System Regulation

Getting into the specifics of the treatment plan, the first thing that needs to be done is to dial down the inflammatory response. This can be achieved using probiotics, Vitamins A and D, anti-inflammatory supplements, anti-allergenic diet, and keeping the blood sugar in check.

The other side of this is going to be detoxification. Typically, this is done after bringing down the immune system's over activity. Keep in mind that with an autoimmune disease, something has come into the body that is triggering a response. In the long run, what you really want to do is work with the body and hope the immune system gets rid of this trigger.

You want to do it in a safe way wherein you're not really pushing the immune system too far. Because if you're just going to push the immune system with medication, you could also push the autoimmune response accidentally, which you don't want to do. However, at some point, you want to get the body healthy enough to go through detoxification; a safe and controlled detoxification.

There are many harsh detoxification programs out there like the Master Cleanse, and those 14-day fasting programs. We're not talking about anything like that. We're talking about gentle, safe detoxification protocols.

Chapter 3 - Effective Natural Treatment for Hyperthyroidism

In this chapter, we're going to have an in-depth discussion on controlling hyperthyroidism symptoms naturally with dietary changes and supplements. Also, we're going to outline a more holistic approach to treating the causes and underlying triggers of hyperthyroidism.

Controlling the symptoms and treating the cause of hyperthyroidism is not the same thing. This might be confusing right now. However, we assure you that by the end of this book, it won't be.

In the previous chapters, we attributed Grave's disease to hyperthyroidism. It has been the cause of hyperthyroidism 90% of the time. Of course, Grave's disease is a severely serious illness. And a thyroid storm is a potentially fatal symptom of Grave's disease. However, many presentations of Grave's disease are mild and can be helped with natural medicine.

Endocrinologists will often recommend that patients have their thyroid gland destroyed, either through radiation or surgery. While this needs to be done in some cases, destruction of the thyroid gland is not always necessary. Grave's disease--and the hyperthyroidism it brings--does not always present itself the same way. A textbook case of Grave's disease is when someone is at risk of going into a thyroid storm, has a remarkable inflammation of the thyroid glands, ophthalmopathy, and pre-tibial myxedema.

However, while the aforementioned symptoms are indicative of Grave's disease/hyperthyroidism, many people are not walking around with all of these symptoms. Also, they're not in an immediate crisis where they need to have their thyroid gland taken out right away. The symptoms that are seen most often are tremors, cardiovascular symptoms, increased appetite, weight loss, heat intolerance, and an elevated blood sugar.

In reality, a lot can be done for people with hyperthyroidism. The cause of hyperthyroidism is not entirely unknown. Of course, there's not a single cause of hyperthyroidism which can be reduced. Hyperthyroidism, like any other autoimmune condition, is a multi-factorial problem and requires individualized treatment plans.

There's no single hyperthyroidism protocol for everyone. However, science does have a good idea of what leads to an autoimmune disease, even if that knowledge has not made its way into conventional medical treatments. Toxic medication such as Methimazole is not required and the elimination of the thyroid gland is avoidable.

Auto-immune or Thyroid Disease?

Grave's disease is primarily not a thyroid disease. It is an immune disorder that affects the thyroid glands. Therefore, any therapy for Grave's disease--whether it's surgery, drugs, nutrition, or herbs--that is only focused on the thyroid glands and not the immune system will do nothing to treat the underlying causes.

With this in mind, we have outlined of a two-step approach to treating Grave's disease below:

1. First, we want to control the symptoms of Grave's disease using as many natural therapies as possible, instead of toxic medications. This is because the supplements are not toxic. Ideally, medications can be eliminated altogether. But this, of course, depends on the severity of the case.

2. Once this is done, we are going to start working on the underlying immune system disorder.

Why Use Supplements To Control Symptoms?

Even though using supplements to control Grave's disease's symptoms will not do anything for the underlying immune system disorder, its use is still important. Why? Because first, Grave's disease is just too serious to leave untreated without controlling symptoms in the meantime. Second, the treatment for the underlying disorder usually takes time to work. Eventually, you do want to get the symptoms of Grave's disease controlled by working on the immune system.

Also, the medications for Grave's disease such as Methimazole are very toxic. Natural supplements, on the other hand, are generally not, as long as they are used in a responsible way. In other words, it is really about taking people off of toxic medications and replacing those with non-toxic supplements.

Lowering Medication Doses

So how does one go about lowering their dose of Grave's disease medication? First of all, do not stop taking medications without talking to your prescribing doctor about it. Do not go out and start taking supplements out of the blue, just to stop taking the medications.

Supplements are first added to the medication protocol. Then, if symptoms improve, the patients can go back to their prescribing doctor to lower the medication dosage. The following are examples of supplements for Grave's disease/hyperthyroidism:

Carnitine

Carnitine is more commonly known for its ability to improve energy levels and to assist in burning fat and losing weight. However, it also blunts the action of excessive T3 at the level of the cell receptor. While this doesn't do anything to lower actual blood levels or thyroid hormone, it will make the thyroid hormone you have less active.

What's really interesting is that in the case of normal thyroid hormone levels, carnitine is not suppressive. It only suppresses thyroid hormone action if there's too much thyroid hormone. There are studies that show how Carnitine is helpful in treating Grave's disease with just doses of two and four grams per day.

Carnitine is not cost-effective in its liquid form, but also the more expensive among all the supplements.

Herbs

Lycopus, otherwise known as bugleweed, is really the most well-known herb for hyperthyroidism and Grave's disease. Other herbs that can help control symptoms are Leonurus or "motherwort" for cardiovascular symptoms, and Melisa or "lemon balm," which is traditionally been used for hyperthyroidism specifically.

Selenium

Selenium is a well-known trace mineral often used in detoxification programs and is also a powerful anti-oxidant. However, a study on blood levels show that increased levels of selenium may improve the outcome of Grave's disease.

There was also an Italian study that proved how selenium was helpful for the visual symptoms of Grave's disease. It was by no means a panacea, but it was helpful. And considering that selenium is cheap, readily available, and it is not harmful in typical responsible doses, there is no reason why it shouldn't be used.

Additional Supplements

Another supplement that can be used is lithium. Its use is extremely limited, however, since it is often associated with psychiatry, manic-depression, and all sorts of neurological side effects. Most physicians found out that when they go through the list of supplements that can be used to control hyperthyroidism's symptoms, patients get scared and will want another alternative.

However, the nutritional dose of lithium that will be used for hyperthyroidism cannot be compared to a farmer's suitable dose. In psychiatry, they'll start people out on 600 mg of lithium a day. A nutritional dose is going to be 5 mg or less, maybe even one and a half milligram. 5 mg is less than one percent of the dose that's used in psychiatry.

In psychiatry, they're using a pharmacological dose to really force an effect on the body. A nutritional dose of lithium is really just giving the body a trace mineral which the body uses and needs anyway. It is not dangerous; it is not going to cause all sorts of neurological effects in these nutritional doses.

Supplements such as Vitamins A, D, and E are fat-soluble vitamins that work together to lower inflammation and regulate the immune system. Right now, there are a lot of people who are mega-dosing on Vitamin D since it has been the fad supplement in the last five or six years. Vitamin D is certainly important. However, it works with other fat soluble vitamins especially Vitamins A and K.

What you should be worried about is seeing a lot of illness caused by relative deficiencies of Vitamins A and K, because people are taking so much Vitamin D. And if you really want Vitamin D to be effective, it needs to work with the other fat-soluble vitamins. Vitamin A is extremely underappreciated; it has an effect on the immune system, it improves gastro-intestinal function, it is anti-inflammatory, and it does work along with Vitamin D. With this in mind, it is therefore preferred to take these vitamins together.

Not all aforementioned supplements are going to be needed in every hyperthyroidism/Grave's disease case. Typically, what's only required is the use of minimum support to keep Hyperthyroidism/Grave's disease symptoms in check. Remember, the most important part is balancing the immune system.

However, out of the vitamins that we've discussed so far, Vitamins A and D are the ones that are recommend to be taken. They're extremely recommended because they lower inflammation and they work on the immune system as well.

As far as diet is concerned, it is recommended that people with hyperthyroidism, Grave's disease, or other auto-immune diseases be on an allergy elimination diet. The big offender that we absolutely want to see taken out is gluten. There should be no gluten whatsoever.

Also, artificial sweetener needs to be eliminated from the diet. Grave's disease and artificial sweetener can be a big problem. In addition to this, there are some foods that are beneficial in hyperthyroidism. These are the goitrogenic foods that people with hypothyroidism are told to avoid.

A goitrogen is simply a chemical that's going to make it more difficult for the thyroid gland to uptake iodine; it's going to stop the thyroid from being able to make so much thyroid hormones.

Goitrogenic Foods

The best goitrogenic food is Millet. It is a less commonly known grain that is a powerful goitrogen. Other goitrogenic foods include Broccoli, Cauliflower, Cabbage, Kale, and Turnips.

Homeopathics and Isopathics

Some other therapies in addition to the standard supplements are going to be Homeopathics and Isopathics. We'll put more emphasis on Isopathics since these are very powerful ways to modulate immune system response, plus the fact that not many people know about it in North America.

Isopathics have been used in Europe for many decades. Only a small number of medical practitioners started using these in the United States. An Isopathic is a very diluted amount of intracellular content of either a fungus or bacteria such as Penicillin Notatum or Penicillin Roqueforti, which is actually the exact same fungus that they make blue cheese out of.

So, this is not live fungus. This is dead intracellular contents from the fungus. What this does is it stimulates the immune system. Once the immune system sees this harmless material, it will then trigger a response. The theory of how this works is similar to that of vaccination with the exception of injecting metals or harmful antigens into people.

The nice thing about Isopathics is that you can stimulate the immune system to start going after that things you want it to go after. However, it will do it in a way that will dial down the aggressive immune system response.

So, if someone has an autoimmune disease, you can use Isopathics to calm down the immune system; to get the immune system to stop attacking itself. At the same time, it will help regulate the immune system function to really start going after the things that you wanted it to go after, whether it's a pathogenic bacteria, or subclinical infections.

There are different Isopathics made from different fungus and bacteria, and their use depends upon each patient and their situation. Using Isopathics in conjunction with Homeopathics really helps tailor protocols for someone's specific situation. It also helps to normalize overall immune system function.

So, this is something that should be used in combination with everything else; the herbs, the nutritional supplements, the different functional tests if needed, etc. All these things work together to normalize immune system function and hopefully get to the real root cause of the autoimmune disease, rather than just telling someone that they have to have their thyroid taken out.

Conclusion

We would like to thank anyone who stuck around and read through the entire book. We know that it might seem a lot of information. However, this is really just the bare essentials that you have to keep in mind to understand what Hyperthyroidism is all about and the natural therapies and supplements involved to get rid of it for life.

If you have a colleague, family member, friend, special someone, etc. who is looking for answers about Grave's disease and Hyperthyroidism, and who does not want to undergo surgery or radiation therapy, please do not hesitate to recommend this book. It just might save their lives.

Thank you.

Made in the USA
Middletown, DE
09 February 2020

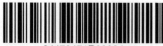